PROTEIN P. 2

"In Shaken but in Control, Paul Ciaravella shares what he has learned, and puts into practice every day, about coping with Parkinson's Disease using natural remedies and a healthy diet. By teaching and promoting this natural approach he has helped so many live a better quality of life."

Janet Matthews
Canadian Co-author
Chicken Soup for the Canadian Soul
Professional Speaker and Spiritual Mentor

SHAKEN BUT IN CONTROL

PAUL CIARAVELLA

BALBOA.
PRESS
A DIVISION OF HAY HOUSE

Balboa Press books may be ordered through booksellers or by contacting:

Balboa Press
A Division of Hay House
1663 Liberty Drive
Bloomington, IN 47403
www.balboapress.com
1 (877) 407-4847

Printed in the United States of America.

ISBN: 978-1-4525-9643-3 (sc)
ISBN: 978-1-4525-9644-0 (e)

Balboa Press rev. date: 5/29/2014

CONTENTS

FOREWORD

Parkinson's disease is on the rise, with more people being diagnosed daily. As of October 11, 2013, there were approximately 60,000 people with this disease, most of them, including myself, don't know how to handle it. I am stepping up to the plate to learn as much as possible about this disease, and to share that information with others, from the perspective of one who has the disease.

Canadians seem to have few answers, yet medications are being prescribed without full knowledge of the long term effects for individuals. These drugs affect individuals differently, and create a variety of challenges with which one has to cope. I believe that a good place to start to take an active role in managing the disease oneself is to make a change in one's own diet, exercise regimen, and overall lifestyle.

Before being diagnosed, life was wonderful in so many ways…being independent, working, spending time with family, enjoying participation in activities with friends, just being. The diagnosis had a tremendous impact. It is up to each individual to be informed and knowledgeable by reading, asking questions, and being involved in the process of decision-making as to programmes of treatment customized to each individual.

I believe that knowledge is a miracle. It creates confidence, and opens up every avenue of opportunity, leaving behind ignorance, leading us on a journey into the unknown. Sickness, a challenge to wellbeing, is always with us, but can be overcome. With faith, alternative solutions can be found. Anger solves nothing; control your anger, or it will control you, and will be a constant threat to your good health and wellbeing.

Keep your family well to reduce vulnerability to challenges like Parkinson's disease, to avoid the costs of ill-health, and to experience the joy of healthy balance and quality of life. That is what is most important!

The Word EDUCATE has its roots in the Latin word "educo," which means to educe, to draw out to develop from within. The best educated man is the one whose mind has been the most highly developed.

May the power of nutrition be with you always.

Paul Ciaravella, author.

CHAPTER 1

ABOUT THE AUTHOR

In 1985, I married Teresa. One year later, our first child, Scotty was born. We lived in the north end of Richmond Hill, better known as Oak Ridges. We purchased our first home, and were a very happy family, with a new baby, two dogs, Harpo and Spock, and two cats, Puss and Boots.

Perry, full of energy, was born in 1987. Our geneticist had recommended a test available to provide early diagnosis of the condition that affected Scotty. Samples were sent to Boston and to the Hospital for Sick Children in Toronto. Although the tests came back negative, Perry exhibited symptoms, similar to those of our first-born, at three months. Perry was diagnosed with the same affliction as Scotty. He passed away five months later. It had been a very challenging beginning to the start of our family.

In May of 1990, I started C.E.S. The outcome of the venture was not what we expected. Getting the business up and running took all of our time, and cash flow became a big issue. There was no time to do research, and everything was a challenge. Matters just got worse as our debt load continued to rise. We had to close the company, sell our house, and declare bankruptcy. We found a house to rent in Maple, just west of Richmond Hill.

Although we were considerably shaken, we were not stirred, and did not get down on ourselves. We discovered that, once committed to a challenge, it was impossible to hold us back. Others may have become shaken over nothing, but we decided to take control and became positive as we focussed on our mission. In the book, Looking Out for Number One, by David Ringer, he talks about South Africa and mining for diamonds. Approximately 2000 pounds of rock and dirt have to be processed to find one diamond.

The average person would give up after the first 100 pounds. It is so important to stay positive, shaken but in control. My 'downs' seem to have outnumbered my 'ups', because there seem to have been a lot of rejections when I ask for something. It has been a learning experience, and I have developed skills to address the negatives, rather than ignore them.

Recently, I ran into a dear friend, David Richard, who introduced me to a new venture. One of the network companies promoted soap. Another sold pet food, but only lasted two years. I did make good connections with good people, and kept in touch. In 1994, one of these contacts, Kim, called to inform me that Marc had started a new company, a wellness company. As I had other things on the go, I asked her to call me in a few months; she called every week for six months. I finally said I would listen to what she had to share. Kim had done a cleanse system, and her health had improved considerably. She suggested that I try it, as I knew little about cleansing the body and rebuilding it at the same time.

During the cleanse process, I lost five inches from my waist, realized an increase in my energy, and saw a new direction in improving my life. The call from Kim opened a door to a network of tutors, who taught nutrition courses, and increased my faith and belief in myself. One such course was promoted in the Richmond Hill paper. Danielle, the instructor was a brilliant nutritionist, and directed me to take a correspondence course offered by David Roland. The cost was $2000, and well worth it; the school offering the course, Canadian Holistic Nutrition, has expanded to southern Ontario. The quality of the educators is exceptional.

In 1995, I met the herbalist of the millennium, Hamad Aboukhazzal, although I call him Yoda. He taught me about herbalism which dated back to the time of Cleopatra, and along the lineage, one child has been taught to pass along the wisdom and knowledge of foods and herbs. Then, I met a naturopath, Ross Anderson, whose teachings were intelligent and easy to understand. Other exceptional individuals in the field included: Dr. Doris Rapp, or the Wizard of Oz of chemicals, as I have dubbed her, with knowledge of cosmetics and chemicals; Dr. Bernard Jensen, a most knowledgeable nutritionist, author of numerous books on the subject of nutrition, and to him I owe my 'black belt in nutrition'; Joel Robbins, a naturopath with nutrition tips to offer from every angle; Elaine Gottschall wrote a book on Crones Disease, focussing on how to break the vicious cycle of the condition. I continued to meet more specialists: Doctor Coon shared that indigestion is connected to arthritis, as digestion has to occur for nutrients to get into the body; Judy Vance wrote a book titled "Beauty to Die For", about cosmetics and the chemicals that are being absorbed into the body; Weston Price's book, "Degenerative Nutrition, explains how children have to wear braces today due to poor nutrition, using research from Francis Pottanger, a dentist who used 'junk food' to experiment on the teeth of cats and dogs during the 1930's.

There are numerous other professionals I met, all sources of information. In the year 2000, I realized that, although I had made significant progress towards my goal of gathering and sharing research, there was still a long way to go.

Financial challenges still exist, with Teresa being the family's sole source of income. Family and friends don't comment, but their faces say it all. I did go back to work, getting a job at the Sears warehouse for a year, qualifying us for a mortgage, which allowed us to purchase a townhouse in 2002, and we still call it home. My knowledge of nutrition continues to expand, resulting in speaking engagements. I created a presentation called "Eat Guilt Free". My first audience numbered 23 guests. Six months later, to an audience of approximately 65 people, I delivered a presentation on foods and GMO's. With the help of Judy Vance and Doctor Doris Rapp, I put together a presentation on chemicals and preservatives in cosmetics. Every guest of the 55 in attendance was impressed, and bought product made with natural ingredients, that was available for purchase after the seminar. When suggesting there is a problem, it is important to offer the solution, rather than just a 'band aid'. With this significant progress, I felt that I was going in the right direction, with greater things yet on the horizon. See picture below explains how problems are easy to solve when you focus on them most people spend 55 minutes worrying about it 5 minutes on the solution I spend 55 minutes solving it and 5 minutes worrying about it.

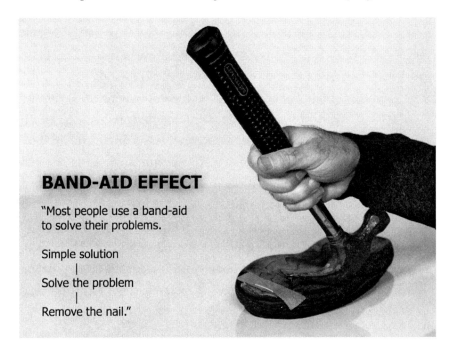

BAND-AID EFFECT

"Most people use a band-aid to solve their problems.

Simple solution
|
Solve the problem
|
Remove the nail."

If you have a nail in your shoe and it is painful easy solution use a ban aid for comfort or remove the nail for permanent solution.

Our bodies consist of many parts, one is the Judge the other is the Jury. The foods that we eat such as Monsanto gmo foods, additives, preservatives pesticides and herbicides are the accused on trial. The Jury are our organs and they determine if guilty or not guilty. My jury called the verdict explaining that this patient suffers from Parkinson's due to the facts he has residues of DDT that are nasty chemicals that were banned many years ago. He also has solvents which come from paints used for thinners.

Furthermore, his blood shows evidence of high levels of lead and pesticides. These chemicals are spreading into the blood and contaminating it.

The jury consists of the heart, lungs, kidneys, small and large intestine, pancreases, thyroid, spleen, skin, eyes, liver, and the brain. Our verdict is ready to be read you're the jury please go ahead with the verdict. Jury please read the verdict due to environmental contamination and pollution to the organs. The Jury finds all these companies and our government NOT guilty which results in the PATIENT IS RESPONSIBLE for his actions. Case Dismissed.

CHAPTER 2

WHAT YOU SHOULD KNOW ABOUT PARKINSON'S

Another challenge was about to present itself.

There are some things you should know about Parkinson's disease before the diagnosis.

I started experiencing lower back pain and went to a clinic in the west end of Toronto. I was referred to a doctor for treatment. Although it was expensive, it produced results. I enjoyed sports, like track and field, especially the 100, 200 and 400 metre sprints, and baseball. My track team nicknamed me "Torpedo", and my baseball teammates nicknamed me "Wheels"; I took it as a show of respect. When I played fastball, I played third base and right field. In slow pitch, I was the pitcher. I had been in good health but, one night, while pitching, I had no elevation of the ball. I could not pitch, and took myself out of the game.

The next day, I had a back treatment with the chiropractor. I told him that I was experiencing tremors in my hands, and he referred me to a neurologist. The appointment with the neurologist was scheduled for two months later. The standard procedures of paperwork and blood work were completed. He scheduled me for an MRI, and indicated that he suspected Parkinson's disease. I asked the cause of the disease, and he distracted me with the comment that the drugs were very expensive. I asked about natural products that might provide relief from the symptoms, but he felt they did not work. I left the office frustrated and furious. The results of the MRI came back negative, but, the following week, results of the blood work indicated evidence of Parkinson's. I returned to his office, where the conversation about expensive drugs and natural remedies was repeated, with the same results of frustration and anger, on my part.

Returning home, I made a few phone calls, only to find that the naturopath solutions were equally expensive. Six months later, with the assistance of a friend, I was able to find a naturopath in Maple. After completing the patient form, he tested for food allergies and bowel inconsistencies, ultimately leading to his suggestion to try chelation.

He also recommended a test performed through the World Health Organization (W.H.O.). Samples of blood and urine were sent, with the readings fairly normal, with the exception of lead levels, which were very high. I trusted the readings to be accurate, as the W.H.O. handled the S.A.R.S. outbreak in Toronto. It was a challenge to determine why the levels of lead in my blood were so high. A number of sources came to mind: During the 1960's, my family owned a gas station that served leaded fuel; each time we moved, the new home was painted, the paint and solvents probably containing lead; Soldering on water pipes in older homes also contained lead.

Additional tests to assess and address my health issues ran at a cost of approximately $400 each. Again the suggestion of chelation was raised, including the additives of Vitamin C and Glutathione, which plays a major role in protecting all cells, especially those in the brain. We elected to go with chelation twice a week for six months, at a cost of $230 per week. The process removed about 5% of the lead, but my energy levels were still very low. Samples of blood and urine were again sent to the W.H.O., headquartered in Atlanta. The results showed the presence of *DDT (dichlorodiphenyltrichloroethane), a synthetic chemical compound, once used widely in the United States and throughout the world as a pesticide.

DDT was in my blood, as well as lead, pesticides and herbicides, DDE, and benzene solvents.

Regulations on the use of dangerous chemicals are more prohibited. However, the presence of these chemicals in the soils is still a threat. There are many challenges to our food sources: Genetic Modification has questionable effects; Golf courses have permission to spray pesticides and herbicides; it is difficult to monitor all agricultural areas on a regular basis.

I believe there is an organic compound that can replace the dangerous chemicals currently in use. It is a mixture of natural minerals, naturally present in the earth. These minerals are similar to ground rocks, as fine as sand, which can be spread on the soil, providing high growth energy. I used 20 bags of this compound on my garden in 2001, and am now reaping the rewards.

even organic

Highest Levels	Lowest Levels
Apples	Asparagus
Bell Peppers	Avocado
Blueberries	Cabbage
Celery	Cantaloupe
Cherries	Eggplant
Cherry Tomatoes	Grapefruit
Collard	Kiwi
Grapes	Mango
Hot Peppers	Onions
Kale	Pineapple
Nectarines	Sweet Corn
Peaches	Sweet Peas
Potatoes	Sweet Potatoes
Spinach	Watermelon
Strawberries	

Lake Ontario

This lake has been polluted over many years. It is important that we pay attention to what we use to wash our clothes, to clean our cars, to wash ourselves. It is also necessary to ensure that we dispose of medications and toxic chemicals safely and responsibly.

Did You Know that...

- a single peanut contains 183 pesticides
- a cup of coffee has over 200 chemicals, including herbicides
- a teaspoon of white sugar shuts down your immune system for 6 hours
- the second ingredient in salt is sugar
- all seedless fruits, like grapes and watermelon, are genetically modified
- a healthy liver takes 12 weeks to process a single deep fried French fry
- English cucumbers, with growth from 2 to 14 inches in a day with the help of chemicals, are grown in hothouses
- we drink our beer cold, because we use low quality ingredients that have a fermentation process of a few days, rather than the 6 weeks that English brews have
- did you know that US farmers currently use approximately 800 million lbs of pesticides and

22 billion lbs of synthetic fertilizer each year and tons of herbicides and fungicides growth regulators fumigants to protect foods while they are in transit and storage. Do the math. Tons of these dumped in the farms environment congratulations you now have Parkinson's disease.

Write to our minister let them hear your voice

Hon. Ralph Gooddale FEDERAL AGRICULTURAL MINISTER House of Commons Ottawa ON K1A0A6

FAX 613 759 1081.

*For more information on DDT, visit www.pesticideinfo.org/ Detail_Chemical.jsp?Rec_Id+PC35419

We have been using pesticides for crops in general since 1874 then we discover DDT in the early 1900 century we started pasteurizing our food like milk then mid 50's the allergies started due to Pasteurizations year 2000 autism is up Parkinson's as well now our water we drink it out of the plastic bottle ignoring the problem in my valued opinion wake up people face it stop caring for your car take care of your colon instead also support your local farmer he might sell you some fresh raw milk.

CHAPTER 3

SYMPTOMS OF PARKINSON'S DISEASE, AND FINDING A SOLUTION

I was diagnosed with Parkinson's disease in 2008. What are the symptoms of Parkinson's, and what is the solution to a cure?

Early symptoms of the disease include:

- Difficulty writing
- Slow movement
- Softer voice
- Feet seem heavy to move
- Hand tremors
- Poor balance when walking
- Drooling
- Always feeling cold
- Challenges with hand dexterity, making it difficult to peel fruit, put a letter in an envelope, hold a cup, dress, shave, hold cutlery

I even noticed tremors in the back of my head when sleeping. Although symptoms can be common to many people, each case is a personal experience. All of this can certainly shake you up, but it is possible to take control, if you choose to learn from the experience. It's not what happens, but what you do about it that counts.

I was initially crushed with the diagnosis. It felt like somebody had pulled the plug, and all the spirit disappeared from my family. My mom, especially, struggled with the diagnosis, and my wife and daughters could not hide their feelings, as the expressions on their faces gave everything away. I was in denial.

The neurologist prescribed medication, and I refused to take it. The family revolted, arranging a meeting at my house so they could strategize as to how to change my mind. It was not pleasant. For 15 years, I had been promoting natural products, and now I was expected to give up on the philosophy and take a prescribed medication. Although I stood my ground, it was an exhausting experience. They finally relented when I said it was unfair that there were so many healthy people against one ailing person. They were shamed into submission.

Pity followed, and that was extremely hard to handle. It was an emotional drain every day, but that is the plight of many who are dealing with serious illness. It is a constant test of strength to stand by one's beliefs, like the use of natural remedies to relieve the symptoms. It didn't help that the majority of my relatives, and those medical practitioners handling my case, did not agree with my philosophy.

The information is certified most of it is personal experience and some of it is researched by me.

Over the years of 2008 and 2009, I struggled more with walking, speaking, maintaining a reasonable level of energy to get through the day; I was feeling close to desperate. Through a friend, I was able to contact a retired medical doctor. I called her office in Aurora, and made an appointment to see her. Debra, the doctor, was not just a retired medical doctor, but had an extensive knowledge about food nutrition and about the value of herbs.

It was a very positive experience, especially as the appointment, scheduled for an hour, ran for 2 hours. Her expertise was such that she was able to determine what foods to avoid and those that would help my situation. The goal was to increase dopamine going to the brain.

Dopamine functions as a neurotransmitter, recognized by nerve cells. Some amino acids, like L-tyrosine, promote dopamine in the brain. Lecithin, found in egg yolks, also promotes dopamine in the brain. The egg yolks also carry 'good' cholesterol. Dopamine is also found in a variety of foods, including: avocado, bananas, bocconcini, coconut oil, egg yolk, fava beans, flaxseed oil, lamb, MCT oil (Medium Chain Triglycerides) oils, mozzarella, olive oil, pumpkin seed oil, raw milk, raw milk culture, turkey, and veal.

The lecithin in egg yolks is very fragile, and is destroyed, along with the 'good' cholesterol, when it is over-heated. It is best to soft-boil, scramble, or eat the egg raw. The oils also lose their value at high temperatures, which also destroys vitamin E and the antioxidant enzymes. Acidity levels increase, reducing it to a free radical. With pumpkin seed oil, at high temperatures, the B complex and vitamins A, K, and E are destroyed.

Minerals, like zinc, iron and selenium survive high temperatures. Zinc plays an important role in the health of the prostate. It also helps to metabolize food, and is key to those who suffer from Parkinson's, as it aids with digestion, promoting faster delivery of dopamine to the brain. Flaxseed oil can be used 3 weeks on and 2 weeks off. Coconut oil can remain stable through the use of high temperatures. It should be certified organic and cold-pressed. Two tablespoons in the morning and in the evening seem to work well. Coconut oil can also be used with oatmeal in protein shakes, in smoothies, in raw desserts, as a spread, as a moisturizer, in soups. In each tablespoon, there are 125 calories, 22% (14g) Fats, 68% (13.5g) Saturated Fat, 0% Cholesterol, 0% Sugar.

MCT oils help to retain lean muscle mass, act as energy source, and are a weight management aid. They are anti-viral, anti-fungal, and anti-bacterial. They are naturally found in coconut and palm kernel oils. They break down rapidly in the liver, and are metabolized differently than other conventional types of fats. They are recommended as a replacement for long-chain fatty acids, when ketone levels as a booster are low. I am using it now, and find the results positive. The change in diet has helped to keep my Parkinson's under control. It is best to avoid foods with high acidity, like refined white flour; these have very little nutritional value.

A friend of mine owns a distribution company, serving bakeries and restaurants. He gave me a tour of his warehouse, 300,000 square feet of white refined flour. The facility is spotless, not a bug in sight. This begs the question, if a bug doesn't want to eat the flour, why would people? People consume tremendous amounts of this refined flour; it is a staple in pasta, bread, pizza, cookies, perogies, doughnuts, muffins, and countless other pastry recipes. As this flour is also high in gluten, it can cause constipation. There are an increasing number of people on a gluten-free diet. Gluten can destroy the villi, located in the small intestine. This leads to Crone's Disease, a very painful and life-changing condition. Alternative choices include rye bread, gluten-free bread, rice pasta, certified organic products. Did you know that the large intestine holds 4 meals; the 5th meal must be eliminated if regularity is to be maintained. Last year in the USA and many previous years the population used twenty thousand tons of laxatives. To me that is a lot of constipation; it seems to me that everyone is constipated in Canada. Nine out of ten people are constipated. There are no numbers on usage of laxatives to date. According to the professionals, death starts in the colon. See back.

What does one do after receiving a diagnosis of Parkinson's Disease? Write down your symptoms, stay positive, surround yourself with positive and supportive people, and stay informed. Suggested reading includes:

How To Be Your Own Best Friend	The Magic of Thinking Big
As Man Thinketh	Vibrant Health from Your Kitchen
Think and Grow Rich	Beauty to Die For
See You at the Top	Guide to Better Bowel Care

The Laws of Success Napoleon Hill	(Pottenger's Cats)
The Bible	learn about juicing , raw foods good fats so on

T he educated man or woman is whose has learned how to get everything he or she needs without violating the rights of his man or woman Education comes within; you get it by struggle and effort and thought .

WHEN YOU DO NOT KNOW WHAT TO DO OR WHICH WAY TO TURN SMILE THIS WILL RELAX YOUR MIND AND LET THE SUNSHINE OF HAPPINESS INTO YOUR SOUL.

DO I USE MEDICATION? OF COURSE.

My neurologist prescribed Levodopa-Carbidopa and Pramipexole two times per day however, they only help a little bit. I know quiet a few people with Parkinson's and their use of these drugs are incredible. In my opinion, I feel that doctors are over prescribing patients their daily dose of medication 5 to 10 times. The average drug user with Parkinson's spends $800.00 per month; I spend $110.00 per month on medicine and I use $ 500.00 a month on organic foods and supplements.

The key is organic foods don't use pesticides and all other non-organic foods have pesticides on them. Unfortunately, doctors are in the dark regarding pesticides because it is easier for them to prescribe medications rather than sit and talk about natural foods and supplements. For me personally, I don't use too much medicine and that has been a success for me thus far. I wrote this book so people can learn which foods do what to our body and how we do and don't benefit from them. Don't be afraid to approach a naturopath or nutritionist to help you. Here are some tips to hire these natural professionals; ask them about Parkinson's, if they know anything regarding the disease, what should I avoid to improve my health as well as life, what foods should I be eating and which supplements are best for me? All you are doing is developing a relation or a trust. Make eye contact; listen to his or her voice carefully to hear if it is solid with no mumbling. Be a good judge, don't be a pessimist. Open your mind and close your wallet. Ask how much they charge. Figure out if they are going to help you or tell you to see a medical doctor.

I have written a whole chapter on foods and supplements which should help you jump start your quality of life as well as do the right thing take your medicine as little possible and learn about foods and supplements, which will help you to enjoy and have a better quality of life.

Not only will you feel better but there is money saved too and this is the theme. "Foods are your best medicine; medicines are your best foods."

I would like to take a minute to talk about one food that works the best for me and it is highly used by the brain. This food is Lecithin. It is found in all nerve and brain tissues which is very rich in egg yolks. When our body lacks Lecithin, our nerves lack strength and the brain becomes weak which makes us become irritable and tired. I have felt this way many times so I made adjustments by adding some more Lecithin to my foods to avoid health challenges. Parkinson's is a shaking disease and I hate shaking so in result I like to control it because nutrients can be depleted by excess mental work and activity business late at night fatigue. There are always lots of things on my mind such as finances, family problems, exposure to extreme weather especially the winter we've had since December 2013. Poor family habits can result in nutrient deficiencies that the brain needs such as protein, fats, glucose, water, oxygen, iron, magnesium, sulphur, silicon, cholesterol, and lecithin as well as a wide range of vitamins. Without these the brain doesn't run as good and the nerves become uneasy. When I eat eggs I soft boil or poach them which doesn't destroy cholesterol and lecithin. By heat, nut butters are very rich in lecithin as well as B Pollen, so don't be afraid to add this to your diet. Oils that rise up to the surface in nut butter jars are pure lecithin, mix it with a spoon or knife. Peanut butter, almond butter, cashew butter, pumpkin seed butter, sesame butter, whole grain cereals, brown rice, millet, rye, yellow cornmeal can be brought to a boil, soaked over night or can be blended raw.

"You get a seed and put it into organic soil with water and it'll be brought to life. Then get the same seed put it into a 400 degree heated oven for a minute then replant it back in the soil. Let me ask you, do you think it will grow? No because it is dead. My point is if you eat just about everything cooked 3 meals per day sensitive foods like lecithin, enzymes and probiotics will be destroyed by the heat. If you do that then come up with a plan to cook your meals differently or go to a health food store and replenish your body."

CHAPTER 4

THE BRAIN

The brain is crucial. It does everything for us: tolerates, rejects, understands, hears, approves, sees, gives insight, sends you messages of fatigue and annoyance, drives your dreams and plans, allows for creativity and logic, gives us balance.

The Brain and Fats

Our brain is 75% fat, and requires fats and oils to function properly. Unfortunately, television commercials and newspaper advertising promote low-fat, low-cholesterol products. This type of advertising is responsible for the 2:00 p.m. fatigue syndrome, when you reach for coffee with cream and sugar, hoping that this will increase the energy level. What actually takes place is that the brain is in need of healthy fats, like a teaspoon of coconut oil or an avocado. The same scenario presents itself later in the evening, about 10:00 p.m., when we go to the refrigerator to find an energy booster. Eating late is a means to getting fat, rather than getting your (healthy) fats. Good fats are fuel, and we need them every day, throughout the day. A list of foods, providing healthy fats, is given in Chapter 2.

I'll Skip Dessert, as It Probably Contains Pesticides

Eating organic is the way to go, as it is the only way to be more certain of what is being consumed. If the water is not filtered, we are the filter; if the air is not filtered, we are the filter. It is important to note here that a cigarette contains 4000 different chemicals, most of which are pesticides.

Apples contain 15 different pesticides, absorbed through spraying. Those contaminants are baked into a pie with the apples. I'll pass on dessert. GMO's can be dangerous, especially as we don't know all the effects, as research is limited. Given that the brain absorbs so much of what we consume, it is no wonder that mental issues seem to be more prevalent.

Where Can You Find Organic Foods

More farmers are growing 'clean' crops, fruits and vegetables free of pesticides and herbicides. Supermarkets are stocking certified organic products, locally grown. Produce grown in hothouses should be avoided, as they are devoid of minerals. More communities are organizing Farmers' Markets. Specific locations of markets include: The Village Market at Bathurst St. and Rutherford Road, open Saturdays from 8:00 a.m. to 1:00 pm; the Dufferin Grove Market at Dufferin St. and Bloor Ave., open on Thursdays from 3:00 p.m. to 7:00 p.m.

How Do You Know It Is Organic

Foods that are organic have certain characteristics:

- Vibrancy of colour apples have brown spots
- Fresh aroma they smell good
- Irregular shapes tomatoes are crocket
- Smaller size my peppers are tiny compare from stores

- The occasional bruise
- A memorable flavour

One of the Key Antioxidants

Glutathione is working for me. The research I have done is worth the time put into it. Glutathione is a master detoxifying molecule key antioxidant. It helps in the prevention of disease in our bodies. Our bodies, with age and stress, are able to produce it. The degeneration of soil quality decreases the quality of the nutrients in produce, creating imbalance in the body's production of Glutathione.

Our environment and free radicals play a negative role in our health. Glutathione is a positive. It has the component of sulphur, considered the heating element. If you are cold all the time, eating certain foods can help: asparagus, avocado, broccoli, cauliflower, cinnamon, figs, garlic, kale, leeks, lima beans, oats, onions, peaches, tomatoes, and turmeric. Too much sulphur can, and will, heat up the body to the point where you feel too hot. Balance can be established with foods like cucumbers, lettuce, mixed greens, Swiss chard, and watermelon.

Milk Thistle helps support the liver. Add this to your diet one month on, one month off. Detoxifying the liver helps. Beets are also a good liver cleanse. Many customers report positive results.

Glutathione is important in managing Parkinson's disease:

- It recycles antioxidants
- It aids in the consumption of sulphur-rich foods
- It helps the body absorb alpha lipoid acid, the brain's second-best friend and important to cells and control of blood sugar

To boost levels of glutathione, take a 30-minute walk daily, take additional supplements of the B complex, and add B12, C, E, enzymes and pro-biotics.

The body has a blue print inside, and knows how to heal itself; it just needs the right tools.

The Glutathione Diet

This diet boosts the level of glutathione in the body, and helps with weight management.

Include the vegetables listed above. Include a 7-oz portion of protein lamb or turkey. Get carbohydrates from oatmeal, rice bread, and wild rice pasta. Drink water with snacks, and include probiotics with every meal. Include fruits like apricots, avocado, figs and peaches. A simple dessert can be made with corn meal, oats and a tablespoon of honey. Drink teas like pau darco, hawthorn, ginseng, and dandelion root.

Every day, I boost my glutathione with these foods, and supplements. Every individual is unique and responds differently to various foods. A health professional can help you find your balance.

CHAPTER 5

KNOW THE CHEMICALS IN THE PRODUCTS YOU USE

If you have Parkinson's, this chapter is a 'must read'.

We all use creams, shampoos, soaps, dish detergents, perfumes, fragrances, shaving creams, hair gels, lipsticks, after shave lotions, toothpastes, deodorants, sun tan lotions, hair colouring products, mouth washes, moisturizers, and the list goes on.

Did you know that a woman, during her lifetime, uses 4 to 5 pounds of lip stick? Is that a good thing? No, as lipstick contains several hundred chemicals. Shampoos contain sodium laurel sulphate, which irritates hair roots. Sometimes, the hair falls out, but remains in the scalp, as in my case. I wonder if it contributes to Parkinson's.

Isopropyl alcohol, used in creams to dry up the skin, is used to avoid that greasy, unwashed look at work. However, after use over two years, the skin looks dry and wrinkled. The cycle continues as a moisturizing product, which also contains isopropyl alcohol, is needed to restore the skin to its original moisture level. Hand sanitizer contains the same chemical, and is used by everyone. In the hospitals, nurses can use a hand sanitizer up to 40 times per shift. Over-use can cause arthritic symptoms to develop. Milk thistle can be used to balance the chemistry. It is important that those diagnosed with Parkinson's keep informed and knowledgeable.

Propylene glycol is found in creams, in children's cereal as a preservative, and in numerous other products. A disturbing fact is that it is also used to degrease engines. Imagine putting a product to degrease engines on your face or on your cereal. Other dangerous chemicals used in foods are BHA and BHT (butylated hydroxy toluene), which is added to fats and cheese products, purportedly to maintain freshness. This is allowed by our Government, in spite of the fact that it is related to causing cancer. We all must be diligent in knowing the food we eat.

Methyl PARABEN is a chemical found in perfumes. There are hundreds of these, each one with a different fragrance. People react differently to excesses of these fragrances: a choking sensation, dizziness, difficulty speaking, nausea, etc. These fragrances are found everywhere in our environment: shopping malls, schools, municipal buildings, churches, office buildings, etc.

Anything you smell goes directly into your lungs and into your blood stream to flow through your entire body, including the brain. What is the origin of Parkinson's, and do these chemicals contribute to it in any way?

While in a pharmacy picking up a prescription, I noticed a number of items on the shelves, including a liquid vitamin supplement for children. It contained methyl PARABEN, and a litany of other chemicals foreign to the vocabulary of the average person. The mouth wash contained propylene glycol as a preservative. There were also 'fillers' that were certainly not contributing to good health.

Chemicals are an enemy that surrounds us. They are common in many households: ant traps and mouse traps; insect sprays and pesticides; cleaning solvents to remove and to clean the car, furniture, floors, toilets; dish soap, laundry soap, air fresheners; paints, engine degreasers, glue, dry-cleaning products.

These products have a smell to them, going into your lungs and the blood stream, causing acute headaches, nausea, and severe dizziness. Some of these products enter the body through the skin, causing irritation and symptoms similar to those chemicals absorbed through the nasal passages. There are also chemicals in the materials of the clothes we wear. Some of these chemicals contain heavy metals, with severe adverse reactions for people diagnosed with Parkinson's. Do the research to find natural products to meet your needs.

Mercury is found in the fillings in your teeth. This affects the immune system, and should be removed immediately in those suffering with Parkinson's. The positive results can be realized within a year for many. It takes time for the body to heal itself; and, like a car, if it is maintained well and powered with the right fuel, the body will run smoothly. We need food free of chemicals, coming from clean soils and fresh water. Much of our produce is grown in greenhouses, and nourished with chemicals. This has been a practice for over 50 years.

Do you drink water? We live in a country with the largest supply of fresh water in the world. Mineral water is a popular choice of bottled water. I was able to 'muscle test' mineral water, and did not find any minerals in it. A good marketing programme can sell anything. Bottled water has replaced coffee and soft drinks at the top of the beverage list. There is a great deal of confusion as to how much water individuals should drink. Some suggested amounts are: 500 ml for children aged 3 years; 700 ml for children aged 8 years; 1000 ml for children aged 12 years (If they are involved in sports, add another 250 ml.); 1500 ml for teens and adults, adding 250 ml for added activity. If one is taller than 6 feet, or doing a detoxification programme, drink 2.5 litres. It is better not to drink water with your meals, as it causes the loss of important enzymes; drink water only between meals. Those with Parkinson's should drink at least 1.5 litres daily.

We breathe in oxygen and breathe out carbon dioxide. Nature has given the body a blue print by which to take care of itself. Cuts heal in 5 to 7 days, as long as the oxygen level of the blood is sufficient. Carbonated drinks lower the oxygen in the blood stream, forcing the body to work harder. The brain needs oxygen. Substitute a smoothie or fruit juice for the carbonated beverages, you'll feel better for it.

YOUR BODY IS LIKE A BARREL

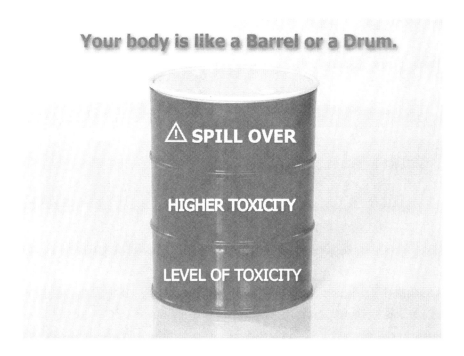

The example made here is about levels of toxins in the body. The first level is acute, which means it is not serious. Level 2 is a higher level of toxins. At this point we have to pay attention to our health as it will show ill symptoms. The spill over happens when toxins reach your blood called auto intoxication.

CHAPTER 6

YOUR BODY'S DEFENCES

Our bodies have a number of warning systems and defence mechanisms. For instance, our feet are very sensitive to heat on the ground, the face and extremities warn us of excess heat and excess cold. One of the symptoms of Parkinson's is that the feet seem to stick to the ground. The reactions of the immune system, the respiratory system, and the digestive system tell us whether we are managing our bodies effectively.

Headaches can be caused by a number of imbalances, one being 'dirty' blood. A colon cleanse, based on personal experience, is very helpful. Another solution is to increase the intake of sodium from produce like celery, kale, potato peels, parsley; together they make a delicious soup to restore sodium and calcium levels. Healthy sodium can also be found in the white of an egg, the white of watermelon peel, celery root, apple skins, many fruits, sea salt. Keep the daily consumption of salt to about one teaspoon.

The term "catch a cold" is very common, but, more accurately, we 'eat' a cold. Germs are picked up on our hands and transmitted into the body when we eat; this is why the message of washing hands frequently, using running water, is often heard. It takes time for food to digest, and germs take this opportunity to multiply. A sore throat can be eased by consumption of more water. When we shiver, the body is letting us know that it needs heat. Internal heat can be elevated by the consumption of foods containing sulphur.

Diarrhoea can be caused by constipation, and is the body's way of clearing the system safely by liquefying solid waste. It can be caused by parasites, worms, or even low levels of magnesium. Parasites can be deadly, often entering the body. Foods that are insufficiently washed and/or cooked are a major cause of the spread of parasites. People with weakened immune systems, like those with Parkinson's, are particularly vulnerable. The urge to spit is also a signal from the body letting you know that something is not right. Bloating and gas can be relieved with a colon cleanse, probiotics and enzymes.

Dizziness can be the result of stress, too little sleep, and poor nutrition. Take note of your daily habits and patterns, and events in your daily life that may be causing an imbalance in your routine. Shaking, or tremors, is not necessarily reserved for those with Parkinson's. It is often a reaction to a traumatic experience, like a car accident. Relief can be found in the B vitamins and in Vitamin C.

Skin irritation is common. Itchiness is the body's way of sending the message that it needs more alkalinity, which can be achieved by consuming more vegetables.

The immune system is our first defence. For those with Parkinson's, immune system boosters include probiotics, acidophilus, antioxidants, whole foods, and live foods. To protect your immune system, avoid refined foods like white flour, white rice, white and brown sugars, fried foods, processed meats and cheeses, coffee, smoking, alcohol, overindulgence with carbohydrates, frozen foods, caffeine products, and carbonated drinks.

To maintain good health, practitioners like qualified medical doctors and certified naturopath doctors should be a part of your personal health team.

CHAPTER 7

FINANCIAL IMPLICATIONS

When a person is diagnosed with a debilitating illness or disease, there are financial implications that impact the individual's lifestyle. It is important to develop a plan for sustainability.

The following numbers are based on a family of four carrying a mortgage of $380,000 at 5%. The combined income of the household is $84,300.

Expense Item	$ Cost
Cable	100
Car, Gas	500
Car Loan	300
Car Maintenance	150
Cell Phones	100
Clothes	100
Credit Cards	100
Dentist	50
Entertainment	100
Food	500
Gifts	50
Heat	125
House Maintenance	150
Hydro	125
Insurance, Car	150

Insurance, House	75
Insurance, Life	100
Internet	50
Medications	100
Mortgage	1947
Taxes, Income	300
Taxes, Property	200
Vacation	0
Vitamins	50
Total Expenses	**$5,347**

This financial plan was verified by a professional, and is only an estimate of a monthly plan. Income tax is yet to be determined and deducted from $84,300 to determine accuracy of net income.

Costs continue to increase at a faster rate than incomes. Examples include: housing costs, interest rates on credit cards, bank fees, insurance rates, income and property taxes, fuel, utilities (cable, heat, hydro). There is also that dangerous draw of the 'luck of the draw' with the promotion of lotteries and gaming. Those unexpected costs for driveway and roof repairs, car repairs, replacement of faulty appliances, can drain every penny of savings in a very short period of time.

Money is a necessity, and there never seems to be enough of it. If you don't control it, it will control you. Loans should be avoided whenever possible.

Since being diagnosed with Parkinson's, there is only a single income earner in our family, and that is my wife, Teresa. Our sources of revenue include her position of Vaughan School Trustee, home daycare, and some government assistance at $906 per month to cover medical expenses, medications in particular. There is no coverage for vitamins, alternative medicines, services from a massage chiropractor or osteopathic naturopath. We budget carefully for those expenses. I plan to start my own small business in natural health products and supplements, using the knowledge I have acquired in getting to understand my diagnosis of Parkinson's. The government taxes any revenue over $5000.

A possible case scenario can be seen in the table below:

Function	$ Amount
Annual Contribution	10, 872
Work Allowance	5000
Deduction	0
Extra income earned	8000
Deduction	3000

This is the system Revenue Canada uses. It is important that the Government look at cases individually, to assess needs. More significant financial investment should be made into research to find the causes and cures for debilitating diseases, like Parkinson's.

Laying blame solves nothing. It is necessary to participate in open dialogue among all parties to resolve the many challenges and impacts, of the many challenging diseases affecting more and more of the population, on society as a whole. Dialogue can start by contacting me by email, which is listed on the back page of this book.

Also a web site is listed.

CHAPTER 8

SOIL FERTILITY, NUTRITIOUS FOODS AND SUPPLEMENTS

Consider the items in the following lists.

Nutritious Foods: Legumes, herbal ingredients, vegetables, fruits, soya, juices, home-grown produce, Vegetarian products, 'live' foods, health food, fresh, natural, home-made, natural, Organic, raw

Popular Foods: Spicy, pork, wheat, beef, dairy products, genetically engineered products, Hydroponically-grown produce, boiled, international dishes (Italian, Chinese, French, Indian, Thai, Greek, etc.), barbecued, 'junk', TV dinners, canned, packaged, Sweets, roasted, baked, refined, 'fast', processed, fried, frozen

Natural, unprocessed foods tend to be vibrantly colourful in greens, reds, yellows, purples, oranges. Healthy, fertile soil produces nutritious fruits, vegetables, and herbs. If the soil is nutrient deficient, then what grows in that soil will be nutritionally deficient for consumption by people and animals. Crops should be rotated, and soil should be pesticide free.

Is what you consume natural and organic? Both terms are over-used, and often for the purpose of misleading the consumer. Take heed of the phrase 'buyers beware'. It is up to the consumer to be informed.

its and vegetables tend to have more nutritional value, as cooking often depletes the nutrients in the produce. Raw foods are better for digestion. When foods are cooked, enzymes are destroyed, making it necessary for your liver to manufacture extra cholesterol, which causes serious health issues. As a guideline, follow the 50/50 rule of 50% raw foods and 50% cooked foods.

Indigestion, causing a bloated sensation, affects many people. It is often caused by not chewing the food sufficiently. Chew until the food is nearly liquefied before swallowing. Something to remember is 'Eat your liquids and drink your solids.' If one has a 5 oz. well-done steak, and it is chewed 50 times per bite, and one has an 8 oz. steak chewed 5 times per bite, the 5 oz. has more nutritional value due to the increased enzymes generated by the additional saliva needed in chewing. Digestive enzymes already exist in our bodies. It is important not to drink large quantities while eating, as this interferes with the digestive process. Fast food restaurants offer large drinks with the various meal packages. These beverages flush away saliva. The temperature of a beverage also affects its value; room temperature is best, as the body doesn't have to warm up the beverage before processing it. Avoid beverages like pop and processed juices, which contain excess amounts of sugar, as this alters the PH balance. As always, be an informed consumer, especially when diagnosed with serious health problems, like a neurological disease.

A sluggish colon is unhealthy. Foods, not completely digested, can build up in the colon. I t is more difficult for the body to break down processed foods. In researching this area, I found that 9 out of 10 people suffer from some form of constipation, with varying degrees of severity and seriousness. Some of the symptoms associated with constipation include headaches, bloating, heart burn, bad breath, body odour, feelings of hunger, sugar cravings, low energy, mood swings, and low libido.

I learned a great deal from my tutor, Dr. Bernard Jensen, Mr. Colon himself, who has written numerous books on the topic, and about nutrition in general. He explains that your bowel can hold four meals, the fifth has to go, 'as the bases are loaded and there is nowhere to go'. It takes about 12 to 14 hours for food to work its way through the digestive system. If it takes longer, then you have a problem to be solved. You may be shaken by the situation, but take control of it. Laxatives are not the ideal solution, as it makes the body lazy. Change the diet. Colours of our fruits and vegetables are significant: greens provide calcium and magnesium; reds stimulate the organs; yellows are natural laxatives. When you make a salad, create a rainbow of the three colours.

Coffee enema can be good for the colon, but coffee, in general, is not advised. The caffeine interferes with the nervous system, and can make shakes worse. Coffee washes out Vitamin C and the B-complex vitamins, leaving dopamine levels low, increasing the magnitude of the shakes. Coffee can also contain residues of herbicides and pesticides, used on the plants during the growing season of the beans. Replace coffee with herbal teas or fresh juices.

Since our soil is not necessarily rich in minerals, it is necessary to include effective vitamin and mineral supplements, especially when dealing with Parkinson's. Additions to your daily regimen should include: major minerals, trace minerals, macro minerals; Vitamin D3; super food green complex; pure phytoplankton; B12, Q enzyme10, B complex; E C A; Daily complete is a liquid botanical which contains 194 vitamins and minerals for dealing with the low energy level symptomatic with Parkinson's; coconut oil, MCT oil, pumpkin seed oil, olive oil which are all organic; to cleanse the body, use a herbal product called Experience, which is the best of the best for the bowel; Vitamin 3D, Vitamin E; Clear (am), Chlorella, Lecithin, Omega 3 Seal Oil, I-tyrosine, maca for men; oil of oregano, cinnamon, probiotics, enzymes.

Seek guidance from a naturopath to determine a daily regimen that works best for you.

We talked about very many foods very many supplements very many fats and oils that do wanders in the body almost saying a cure or a heal I am making no false statements these are some of the personal experience you should be aware that the body heal it self no claims are made .

"Your health is a gift you earn your diseases I graduated with Parkinson's what about you"

Paul Ciaravella, nutrition counsellor.

CHAPTER 9
EXERCISE AND ATTITUDE

If you have been recently diagnosed with Parkinson's, this chapter offers some tips regarding management of the disease through exercise and attitude.

Exercise helps! One of the easiest exercises to do is walk. Other effective options include yoga, Tai Chi, and cycling. A chart of some simple stretches is included in this chapter. It is also important to maintain a positive attitude. Everyone needs to feel positive and good about him/her. Exercise makes it easier to develop that positive attitude.

Some of the items you need to start your exercise regimen are: a stationary bicycle, a yoga mat, a floor mat, abs equipment, light weights, a large exercise ball, and a rebounder.

Mental fitness is also important. Make sure you have a chess set, a checker set, and include some mind fitness games. Part of mental fitness is developing a positive attitude. Socially, some people find it difficult to interact with those with Parkinson's, or any other health challenge. Think beyond the obstacle. Read informative and positive material. Watch upbeat television programming. Turn negative conversation around to the positive. Create a wish list of dreams to make a reality. Exercise your brain with simple activities, like creating a list of opposites: up and down, high and low, rich and poor, heavy and light, etc. This kind of activity targets the left side of the brain, and creates a feeling of being refreshed.

Take note of your level of confidence. You need to manage attitude, just as you manage diet and exercise.

MENTAL EXERCISE list of opposites

Hot	cold
Dark	bright
Fat	skinny
Rich	poor
Heavy	light
Big	small
Good	bad
High	low
Weak	strong
Wide	narrow
Hot	cold
Wet	dry
Smooth	rough
Hard	*SOFT*
Fast	*SLOW*
Fit	*UNFIT*
Black	*WHITE*
Full	*EMPTY*
Positive	*NEGATIVE*

I left some for you to do there are over 1 hundred of these opposites find them and exercise your brain.

Explore new area new territory of your brain learn another language this forces the brain to go to another section another territory new frontier this is so important Doctors are ignoring this area all they are interested in their drugs to them it is the only solution.

Learn about music this is an area of expanding the brain more territory will be used, new songs get involved enjoy your self.

Dancing is also brain stimulant you get to practice balance and music both good normal people too it is good for every body watch young people they love this area of life.

I was talking to a friend of mine some time ago. He has a music school in the Maple area and was telling me how his students benefit, from dancing and learning music their math has improved school grades are better over all parents are happier school teachers their job is easier.

My wife often does church fund raiser there is food music often held in a church hall the people are mixed 50 60 70 older crowd when they go home their smile is above the norm music and dancing has something to do, so try it what do you have to lose.

Knitting is also a great way to stimulate the brain. This being because all the work is done with the fingers. So, playing pool is another each move requires a different angle shot. Playing the piano also is good practice your fingers are controlled by the brain should you have extra dopamine in your brain you will be able to play the drums so engage in some of these along with nutrition water filter and the proper supplements I do most of these before I couldn't half of my life is back.

CHAPTER 10

FOODS RECOMMENDED BY OTHER PEOPLE

We are bombarded with information from Marketing Boards and Fast Food Chains, and through promotional material like the Canada Food Guide, and private organizations. There are often conflicting studies, like those studies on wheat and gluten.

It is the responsibility of Marketing Boards to promote products under their jurisdiction: dairy, beef, eggs, soya, corn, wheat, pork, bananas, and oranges. The consumer relies on the due diligence of the producers and marketers to provide accurate information in a responsible manner, with the best interests of the consumers in mind. More and more consumers are taking it upon themselves to research information as to the quality of the products they are consuming. The organic movement is growing, as many question the dangers to health from fertilizers, pesticides, and herbicides used on crops, and from antibiotics and steroids used on livestock. Much research is being done as to how the consumption of these additives, through the food we eat, affects our health as it relates to cancer, Parkinson's, and heart issues. The best scenario is to be an informed consumer; ask the questions.

There are many contradictions:

- Calcium in milk is healthy; but there seems to be an increase in the number of people with milk allergies.

- Protein is good for us; but much of our meat comes from animals that are given antibiotics and/or steroids.
- Eggs are very nutritious; but the chickens are often raised in cages and fed medications, and the time between the laying of the eggs and the consumer's purchase of the eggs raises concern.
- The Vitamin C to be found in oranges is often compromised because the oranges are picked before they are fully ripe to allow for shipping time. Bananas present a similar problem as it relates to potassium levels.
- The level of iron, used as a promotion for purchasing spinach, is not as high as we are led to believe.
- Corn crops are under scrutiny because of genetic modification. Long term effects are yet to be determined.

Canada's Food Guide attempts to offer information so that the consumer can create a healthy diet, based on food groups and serving sizes per individual. The consumer must keep in mind that these are guidelines only. Each individual is different, and should pay attention to how their own chemistry reacts to foods consumed. Information and education are vital for good health. The consumer must keep in mind that all levels of government have responsibility to generate economic growth. The steadily increasing population on the Earth is raising concerns as to the sustainability of our food sources. There are many challenges to overcome to ensure that the food available will contribute to good health for all people.

Canada's Food Guide suggests:

- Fresh, frozen, or canned vegetables, ½ cup daily
- Leafy vegetables, ½ cup daily
- Raw vegetables, 1 cup daily
- Bread, 1 slice
- Bagel, ½
- Flat bread, ½

Cooked rice, ½ cup
- Cereal, ½ cup
- Cooked pasta, ½ cup
- Milk, 1 cup
- Canned milk, ½ cup
- Yogurt, ½ cup
- Kefir, ½ cup
- Cheese, 1½ oz
- Fortified soya beverage, 250 ml
- Cooked fish, 1 cup
- Shellfish, 1 cup
- Poultry, 2½ oz
- Cooked legumes, 175 ml
- Tofu, 175 ml
- Eggs, 2
- Peanut butter, 30 ml
- Shell nuts, 60 ml   NO   NO   NO
- Oils – canola, olive, butter, soybean, shortening, margarine
  SESAME   COCONUT

Governments are often influenced by Marketing Boards and Consumer organizations. Whatever we consume plays a significant role in the quality of our physical and mental health. It makes sense, especially economically, to have a healthy population. Our food sources have to be reliable, and information has to be accurate.

Alkalinity in the body is very important to good health, and is a defence against disease and death. The following lists, from Ragnar Berg of Germany, indicate foods creating alkalinity in the body and those generating acid in the body.

Column 1	Column 2	Column 3

Alkaline-Forming Non-Starch Foods:	Alkaline-Forming Proteins and Fruits:	Alkalin Starchy
alfalfa, artichokes, asparagus, beans (string), beans (wax), beets (whole), beet leaves, broccoli, cabbage (red), cabbage (white), carrots, carrot tops, cauliflower, celery knobs, chicory, coconut, corn, cucumbers, dandelions, eggplant, endive, garlic, horse-radish, kale, kohirabi, leek lettuce, mushrooms, okra, olives (ripe), onions, oyster plant, parsley, parsnips, peas (fresh), peppers (sweet), radishes, rutabagas, savory, sea lettuce, sorrel, soy beans (products), spinach, sprouts, summer squash, swiss chard, turnip, watercress	dates, figs, grapes, grapefruit, lemons, limes, oranges, peaches, pears, persimmons, pineapple, plums, prunes, raisins, rhubarb, tomatoes **Acid-Forming Proteins and Fruits:** beef, buttermilk, chicken, clams, cottage cheese, crab, duck, eggs, goose, fish, honey (pure), jello, lamb, lobster, mutton, nuts, oysters, pork, rabbit, raw sugar, turkey, turtle, veal, all berries, apples, apricots, avocados, cantaloupes, cherries, cranberries, currants	bananas (sweet), potatoes (white), pumpkin, squash **Acid-Forming Starchy Foods:** barley, beans (lima), beans, (white), bread, cereal, chestnuts, corn, cornmeal, cornstarch, crackers, grape nuts, gluten flour, lentils, macaroni, maize, millet rye, oatmeal, peanuts, peanut butter, peas (dried), rice (brown), rice (polished), roman meal, rye flour, sauerkraut, tapioca

⌐ombine foods from columns one and two, and also from one and three. Avoid combinations from columns two and three.

Learn to balance your blood. Our blood is 80% alkaline and 20% acidic. We need to learn about portions, and the 6-2-1-1 formula:

6 vegetables	60%
2 fruits	20%
1 protein	10%
1 carbohydrate	10%
Total	**100%**

The above information is taken from **Vibrant Health Book** by Bernard Jensen.

Fast Food Guides are available because we are a society on the run. The way we eat causes health problems. More time needs to be taken to eat our food properly and have it digest effectively. Millions of dollars are spent on health care associated with unhealthy eating habits and patterns. It is necessary to eat the right foods in the right way.

Wheat and gluten have become topics of discussion, as intolerances to both seem to be on the rise. Our society consumes large quantities of products containing wheat and gluten: bagels, pastries, cookies, muffins, perogies, pastas, waffles, toast, pizza, oats, panzerotti, pancakes, doughnuts, gravies, breads, croutons, cereal, patties. The overuse of gluten is a widespread dietary issue, as it creates low blood calcium and other minerals, both of which are necessary for the health of organ tissue."

"Taber's Medical Dictionary says that "Celiac Disease is intestinal malabsorption caused by a substance in gluten and characterized by diarrhoea, malnutrition, bleeding tendency and hypoglycaemia. Treatment is a gluten-free diet, perhaps continued indefinitely."

"Gluten causes inflammation, then damages the bowel wall leading to extreme malnutrition, starvation and chemical depletion. Extreme losses of iron, calcium, magnesium, and Vitamins A, D, and E have been noted in the research of Drs. J. F. Phillips, G.L.D. Bensen, J. A. Blaint, and S. Goldman. Celiac Disease may appear at any time during a person's life, and the only effective treatment yet found is a gluten-free diet, including removal of all wheat, which is a heavy gluten food used in great excess in the U.S."

Those suffering from Parkinson's should eliminate gluten foods from the diet.

The above information comes from the book, **Vibrant Health from Your Kitchen** by Bernard Jensen. It is, in the opinion of this author, one of the most informative and knowledgeable books on nutrition available. It is a worthwhile addition to anyone's library.

There are many natural remedies, and food and cooking tips to improve your health. Again referring to Dr. Bernard Jensen's book, **Vibrant Health from Your Kitchen**, pages 250 through 300 have many valuable food tips and remedies. There are many recipes and ideas to help you create a plan for good health: salads, soups, protein and vegetable dishes, egg recipes, vegetable dishes, teas, fruit cocktails, desserts health breads; as well as hints for cooking foods, kitchen hints, freezing and drying foods, body hints; and information on a key to acidic and alkaline foods. It has proven to be a very valuable resource for me, and can be ordered through me or directly from California.

Just as important as the food you consume is the product in which you prepare that food. Cooking should be done in stainless steel, which remains stainless after use and keeps its shine. A good test for the quality of your stainless steel is taking a magnet and placing it on the surface of your pot. If the magnet sticks, it is not a quality stainless steel. Throughout the world, stainless steel is made in a number of countries. Stainless steel has 2 alloys, nickel and chrome, the ideal balance of which is 18/10. The ratio of the two components, for various countries making stainless steel is: Italy, Germany, and England – 18/10; South America and India – 18/8; China – 18/6."

CHAPTER 11

ELECTRO MAGNETIC IMPACT

There is increasing concern about the effects of electro-magnetic waves on the health of all living creatures.

Items transmitting, or using, these waves, include: cell phones, computers, new light bulbs, wireless technology, WI-FI technology, cell towers, clock radio alarms, laptop computers. The increase in the use across the globe is enormous.

The average consumer is relatively ill-informed about how new technology works, and its impact on our physical and social health. This author believes that electro-magnetic waves negatively impacts his health, already in crisis with Parkinson's.

You may find the following resource helpful:

Andrew Michrowski, Ph.D.
The Planetary Association for Clean Energy, Inc.
100 Bronson Avenue, Suite 1001, Ottawa, ON K1R 6G8
Telephone: 613.236.6265
Fax: 613.235.5876 or 6265
Email: paceincnet@gmail.com
Website: www.pacenet.homestead.com

CHAPTER 12

THE BEST OF ME

As I travelled throughout Ontario, particularly in the Greater Toronto Area, and in the United States, I met many people and learned a great deal. While in England, where I actually had my appendix removed, I realized that doctors, as professionals, have many similarities. The most obvious one is that they all want to help people. Whether in San Diego, California or at a conference in Phoenix, Arizona or at a convention in Toronto, Ontario, doctors wanted to improve the health of their patients.

I started my journey with doctors on a mission dedicated to my first two infants. It began with 100 doctors at Toronto's Hospital for Sick Children. It seems to me that all my experience and research has led me to believe that the first solution to health issues is a healthy lifestyle through exercise and a healthy diet of foods grown in soil free of pesticides and other contaminants, and meat from animals raised in a free range environment and free of steroids and antibiotics. Medications to our ailments are a short-term easy solution, but not a sustainable one.

There are four body types: cold, hot, damp, and dry. This I learned from a Master Herbalist studying remedies going back to the days before Cleopatra.

Cold bodies feel vulnerable in cold weather. With Parkinson's, I struggle with the cold. In many households, the heat setting can be a topic of contention among the family members. 85% of women have a cold body type. A number of reasons explain the phenomenon of cold bodies: DNA

structure and genetic foundation, diet, level of mobility
circulation. It is easy to recognize the individual with a (
need for extra clothing and bedding, cold feet and hands, a
temperatures, distaste for winter weather. Foods that can   ⌐ool
body temperature include lettuce, cucumbers, some fruits, green beans,
watermelon. Foods that can generate body heat include onions, garlic,
cayenne, asparagus, broccoli, kale, leeks, figs, lima beans. These 'hot' foods
contain sulphur and can heat up the body. Balance is always important, so
a diet should always be a 50/50 split. To keep the brain cool and to avoid
inflammation, make sure your diet includes probiotics and Q Enzyme 10.

Hot bodies enjoy cooler temperatures of the Fall and Winter months.
85% of men have a hot body type. Some common physical characteristics
include wider shoulders, taller height, and defined jawline. For these body
types, sweating is an issue during the Spring and Summer months.

The individual with a damp body type is always complaining that they are
overweight. They also tend to crave a lot of sugars. The damp term means
that there is water weight, so it is necessary to dry up that situation. This can
be done by consuming herbs and vegetables, and avoiding carbohydrates.
To clear the digestive system, add yellow fruits and vegetables to the
diet: beets, peppers, beans, mangos, peaches, squash, carrots, tomatoes,
potatoes, cornmeal, and alfalfa tablets. Also, as mentioned in Chapter 10,
use the 6-2-1-1 balance for the blood,.

The dry body type tends to not have weight issues. Characteristics of this
body type include dry skin, high metabolism, and healthy appetite.

Regardless of the body type, serious health issues are, in some way,
connected to, and exacerbated by, our environment. In my next book, "I
am certified organic, are you?", I will address ways to improve.

ENDORSEMENTS

My sincere appreciation goes to the following individuals for their support and kind words of endorsement. (Paul Ciaravella, author of Shaken but in control

I can't believe how much knowledge Mr. Paul Ciaravella has devoted to his cause. (Michael Schmidt, Glen Colton Farms)

I have known Paul Ciaravella since 2002. He explained to me about parasites, when I met him originally. Getting to know him was something to wake up for, assuring me that there is somebody out in the field of nutrition with expertise in foods. (Deepica Mital, President and C.E.O, Terra Tree Foods Inc.)

I met Paul Ciaravella in 1997. He has proven to himself that nothing is an insurmountable challenge. He is a powerhouse of knowledge. I am glad to know him, recognizing what a challenge Parkinson's has been. (Robert Azzopardi)

I have known Paul Ciaravella for 15 years, through the Organic Waldorf Market. He is a nutrition counsellor, explaining the importance of supplement, probiotics, and DETOX. He is very knowledgeable, professional, dedicated and active in the field. I wish him the best of luck with his new book. (Mayda Bach, Nutrition Counsellor)

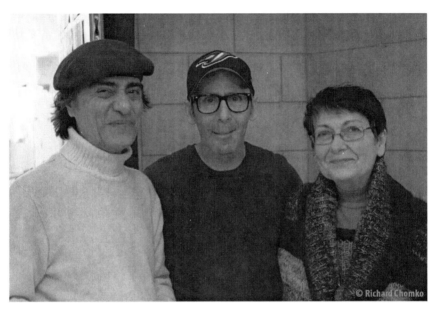

Pictured above: Jack, Paul, and Mayda

ACKNOWLEDGEMENTS

I would like to thank the following professionals for their input:

Hamad Aboukhazaal, Master Herbalist, source of knowledge, experience, and wisdom

Deborah A. Drake, B.Sc., M.D. (retired), N.H.P., CBS., food and chemistry expert

Elaine Gottschall, author of **Breaking the Viscious Cycle**

Dr. Bernard Jensen, author of **Vibrant Health from Your Kitchen**

Dr. Doris J, Rapp .M .D, FAAA,FAAP, cosmetic and food allergy expert

Michael Schmidt, knowledgeable farmer

Dr. Mark Tahiliani, N.D., herbs and food expert

Judy Vance, author and cosmetics expert

David Roland P H D nutritionist (Corola Barzak nutritionist)

Eric Marsden, BSC, ND

Dr Lisa Markson, MD, F.R.C.P.C. Neurologist

Richard Chomko - Photography

CNTO Studios - Photography

Link to supplements:
www.nocravings.puretrim.com

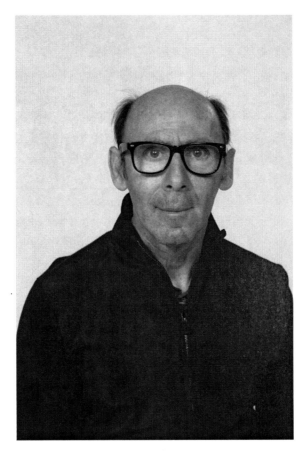

Paul Ciaravella, Author
purejoyhealth@yahoo.ca
www.paulciaravella.com

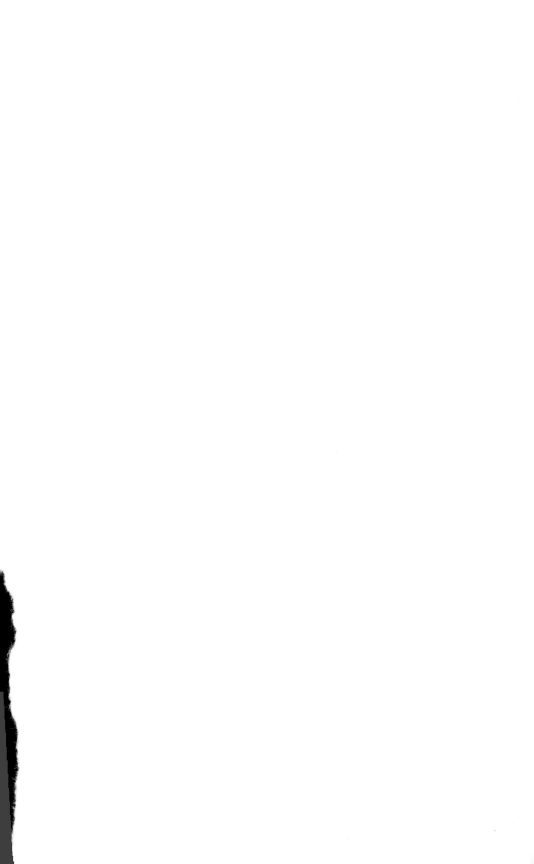

CPSIA information can be obtained at www.ICGtesting.com
Printed in the USA
BVOW07s1421090714

358644BV00001B/1/P